I0447740

Sleep

7 Steps To Break The Insomnia Cycle Forever

by Dean Foster

© 2016 Dean Foster
All Rights Reserved

Table of Contents

Disclaimer

While all attempts have been made to verify the information provided in this book, the author does not assume any responsibility for errors, omissions, or contrary interpretations of the subject matter contained within. The information provided in this book is for educational and entertainment purposes only. The reader is responsible for his or her own actions and the author does not accept any responsibilities for any liabilities or damages, real or perceived, resulting from the use of this information.

Introduction

Sleep disturbances can really take a toll on you, and for many of us, sleep medications have side effects that can affect your waking hours almost as much as lack of sleep does.

Yes, sleep medications will put you to sleep, but it can be difficult to wake up and feel alert; and for those with sleep apnea, sleeping pills can wreak havoc.

The best solution for insomnia does not come in a pill bottle, it comes from understanding what is wrong with your sleep patterns, and working to eliminate the problems that are triggering your insomnia.

There are many sleep disturbances that can cause insomnia. It is important to learn about sleep disturbance in general, the more you know, the better you can cope.

Working with these 7 steps will eliminate your insomnia for good, as long as you stick to them and make them part of your sleep routine. Sleep routines can really affect your quantity and quality of sleep.

Insomnia itself can cause multiple health problems and these health problems will get worse the longer the insomnia lasts. Doctors can always treat your symptoms, but treating insomnia from a medical perspective is not always effective.

Pills will only mask the problem, and many sleeping pills are addictive. One of the biggest problems for those who take sleep medications is that they are less effective the longer you take them, your body will build up a tolerance and you will eventually need a stronger or a different medication.

This book focuses on the causes of insomnia and explains how to use 7 steps to break the insomnia cycle forever. Forever is a long time, these steps will work as long as you make the permanent changes necessary.

Insomnia can and will return if you stop using the 7 steps. As long as you use these steps you will be able to banish insomnia when it rears its ugly head.

Each step covers a specific trigger and a unique counter for the trigger. In some instances, you may need to change your diet and your evening routine. These steps deal with 7 triggers, and each step has several unique behavioral and physical counters that can be applied to rid yourself of insomnia whenever it hits.

Some people may only need to employ one or two steps, other may need to go through all of them; regardless, one or more will help you defeat your insomnia.

The steps in this book work together to reset your circadian rhythm. You circadian rhythm is what regulates you wake sleep cycle. If you suffer from insomnia, your circadian rhythm needs a reset too.

Repeating the steps in this book and making them part of your everyday life will help you create a sleep wake cycle that will destroy that insomnia and give you some much needed, refreshing, recuperative sleep.

Chapter 1 – Sleep Disorders from Apnea to Insomnia

Sleep itself is important for your mental and your physical wellbeing. Lack of sleep has many consequences that can make everyday life a struggle. Lack of restful, refreshing sleep is labeled as insomnia; however, many sleep disorders contribute to or even cause insomnia.

It is important to see a doctor if you have insomnia; sometimes correcting a pre-existing sleep disorder will relive the insomnia.

Anything that disturbs your sleep on a regular basis has the potential to cause insomnia. Snoring by you or your partner can cause insomnia; the constant disrupted sleep can eventually disrupt your sleep wake cycle and cause sever bouts of insomnia.

Correcting the snoring will remove the trigger that caused the insomnia, but you may still be left with insomnia itself.

Every sleep disturbance that occurs on a regular basis can trigger insomnia, if the disturbance continues for any period of time, and the insomnia continues, correcting the sleep disturbance may leave you to battle the insomnia it created.

Recognizing a sleep disturbance and correcting it quickly can eliminate the insomnia before it takes hold.

Understanding sleep disorders will help you eliminate triggers before they cause insomnia itself.

Sleep Apnea

Sleep Apnea is a huge problem that can go unnoticed for long periods of time. Two types of sleep apnea exist; central sleep apnea and obstructive sleep apnea.

Central sleep apnea is rare, bouts of central sleep apnea occur when the brain does not send the proper breathing signals and breathing becomes shallow or stops altogether.

Obstructive sleep apnea is the most common form of sleep apnea. Obstructive sleep apnea occurs because the airway restricts airflow because of a partial or complete collapse in the airway. The obstructed air way cuts off breathing and can cause snoring.

Both types of sleep apnea cause the patient to wake up several times during sleep. When the apnea occurs, the individual moves from deep sleep to light sleep because the brain sends wake signals to trigger the person to wake up and take a breath.

Sleep apnea can occur up to 100 times during an hour, the more it occurs the less restful sleep the individual will get.

Each time apnea occurs the body wakes up in an effort to restore the airflow. The constant disrupted sleep can eventually lead to insomnia. If you have apnea, or think you may have sleep apnea, seek a professional's help.

Apnea can be diagnosed through a sleep clinic and there are ways to live with apnea and sleep through the night.

Sleep Paralysis

Sleep paralysis occurs during the transition between sleep and wakefulness and the transition between wakefulness and sleep. During sleep, the brain signals a paralysis of the body to keep the body from moving during dreaming.

When sleep paralysis occurs, the individual becomes aware and awake but the body is still paralyzed. The body can remain paralyzed for seconds up to several minutes.

During sleep paralysis the individual may sense a presence near them, hallucinate, or experience a pressure on the body, as if someone or something is holding them down.

These fearful experiences occur because the mind is not really fully awake and it is still capable of creating a "dreaming" scenario. Individuals who experience these fearful episodes cannot react to them because the body is still paralyzed. This condition is not a serious one, but it is very disruptive to restful sleep.

Parasomnias

Parasomnia means abnormal sleep. There are several parasomnias identified by the medical field, and each one can disrupt sleep and cause a lack of restful, quality sleep. The following are the most common parasomnias diagnosed by sleep doctors.

- Sleepwalking – Sleepwalking or somnambulism is a sleep disorder that causes individuals to get up and walk, and/or perform actions while sleeping.

  This affects 4% of adults and is more common in children. Those who sleepwalk have no memory of what they did while sleepwalking. Sleepwalking occurs during deep sleep/non-REM and leave the individual with no recollection of the event

- REM Sleep Behavior Disorder – This is more common in men aged 50 or over. During an episode of REM sleep behavior disorder, the individual will act out dreams, many dreams are violent in nature.

  This disorder is dangerous for the individual who has it and their sleep partner. The usual paralysis that occurs before REM begins does not occur and the individual is able to act out the actions of the dream.

- Nightmares – Dreams that are reoccurring, realistic, vivid, and frightening are considered nightmares. Most people experience nightmares sometimes, but nightmares become a parasomnia when it disrupts sleep on a regular basis.

- Night Terrors – Night Terrors affect about 3% of adults, it is more common in children. Night terrors occur during non REM sleep, the individual will wake up startled, frightened and disoriented/confused, and they have no memory of why.

- Nocturnal Sleep Related Eating Disorder – This disorder involves an individual who sleepwalks and eats food. This can cause weight gain and is dangerous because the individual is not aware of what they are doing and are at risk of eating nonfood items, and items they are allergic to.

- Bruxism – Bruxism is grinding the teeth. This condition is damaging to the teeth and the jaw. Those who have this condition can break, wear down, and even lose their teeth.

Sleep disorders keep sufferers from getting restful sleep, and they suffer from the effects of disruptive low quality sleep. Many of these conditions are medical and should be treated by qualified sleep doctors. If they are left untreated and undiagnosed their sleep suffers and the conditions can escalate.

All of these sleep disturbances can result in insomnia. Any long term sleep disturbance can lead to insomnia, once insomnia takes hold, it can linger even after the initial sleep disturbance subsides or is treated.

If you suffer from any of these sleep disturbances, it is important to seek treatment for any sleep disturbance. Once the sleep disturbance is diagnosed and treated, any lingering insomnia will respond to the 7 steps in this book.

Chapter 2 – Insomnia and Medical Causes

The sleep disturbances noted in chapter 1 can and do cause bouts of insomnia but there are other causes. It is important to know if your insomnia is caused by an underlying medical condition. Many medical conditions note insomnia as a symptom and some medication can also cause bouts of insomnia.

The steps in this book can help alleviate insomnia brought on by a medical condition or medication only if the medical condition is treated and the medication changed or stopped. It is important to check with your doctor if you suffer from bouts of insomnia or long term insomnia.

Knowing the causes for your sleeplessness can go a long way to returning you to a regular, healthy sleep cycle.

Non-24 sleep – wake disorder is a chronic sleep disturbance suffered by those who are blind or living in an area with an irregular light/dark cycle in nature. The odd light/dark cycle or the inability to see the light/dark cycle can result in a circadian rhythm problem. This causes the person to wake or sleep at the wrong times during the day.

Non-24-hour sleep-wake disorder should be diagnosed because it can result in long term insomnia if left untreated. Treating this condition usually returns the circadian rhythm to normal and if it was treated early enough, insomnia will improve on its own.

Non-24 is just one example of a condition that triggers insomnia; others include:

- Chronic pain

- Asthma

- Hyperthyroidism

- Nasal and sinus allergies

- Arthritis

- Gastrointestinal issues

- Parkinson's disease

Chronic pain makes it difficult for the sufferer to fall asleep and stay asleep. When chronic pain occurs during sleep it will cause the sufferer to wake up; this constant arousal from sleep can cause bouts of insomnia. Reliving the pain for the entire night will go a long way to resolving the secondary insomnia.

Asthma left undiagnosed or untreated can disrupt sleep. When sleep is disrupted several times a night due to asthma, it becomes difficult to fall asleep and stay asleep.

Alleviating the asthma can help resolve the insomnia. Another problem for asthma sufferers is the inhaler. Many inhalers contain stimulants, these stimulants can cause insomnia and disrupt healthy, restful sleep.

Hyperthyroidism is a condition that causes the sufferers system to race. The heartrate increases periodically and the entire system begins to race. Hyperthyroidism is treatable, once treated wake sleep cycles should begin to return to normal.

Nasal and sinus allergies have symptoms that make it hard for a sufferer to sleep and stay asleep. Back drip from the sinus can interrupt sleep and blockage of nasal airways make it difficult to fall asleep and stay asleep.

Medication used to treat allergies and decongest the sinus and nasal cavities can also stimulate the system and make it difficult to sleep. Proper treatment can alleviate the symptoms and help restore normal sleep patterns.

Gastrointestinal problems can and do interrupt sleep. Acid reflux and other issues can keep sufferers awake and make it difficult for them to sleep through the night.

Neurological conditions can cause sleep disturbances and can also trigger insomnia. One neurological condition that can make it difficult to sleep is restless leg syndrome. Those with restless leg syndrome can experience the symptoms of this condition while trying to fall asleep or they may be jarred awake by the condition.

Each condition listed here can trigger insomnia, using the 7 steps without seeking treatment for these conditions will only ease the insomnia, no stop it. Treating these conditions will help resolve the insomnia and the 7 steps will eliminate it completely.

Chapter 3 – Tips for a Better Night's Sleep

Insomnia is not the only sleep problem that can disrupt everyday life. Sometimes it may be difficult to fall asleep and stay asleep but insomnia is not the cause. Insomnia is a condition that persists for days and even months, sometimes something as simple as a stressful day at work or anxiety over a test can make it difficult to fall asleep and stay asleep.

During these times, a few simple tips for a better night's sleep can make a real difference between waking refreshed and ready to go, or dragging yourself through the day, struggling to focus. If you don't have insomnia, but are finding it hard to fall asleep, these tips will help you relax and drift off.

- Learn Yoga – Yoga can help you relax and de-stress, reducing stress will naturally help you fall asleep. Use your knowledge of yoga to reduce stress and relax before bed time.

- No Caffeine – If you are having a stressful day or stressful period of time in your life, reduce your caffeine intake to help reduce your body's reaction to the extra stress.

  Do not use caffeine or stimulants to stay awake and study for tests, set time aside to study and give yourself enough time to unwind after studying before hitting the hay.

- A Warm Bath – A warm bath can relax the muscles and help you unwind from a stressful day. Try using aromatherapy items during the bath, scented oils and candles can also help relieve the stress of the day and relax you.

These tips will not help you beat insomnia, but they will help you achieve a better night's sleep if stress is keeping you awake. Sometimes we just can't turn off the chatter in our minds and worry or stress keep our minds occupied and awake.

Taking time to for yourself to go over the events of your day long before it is time to sleep can help give you a better night's sleep.

Anxiety and depression interfere with sleep, even if you don't have insomnia, anything that interferes with sleep will affect you during waking hours. If you have Anxiety or depression, there are some tips that can help you maintain a healthy sleep schedule.

Tips for Reducing Anxiety

- Limit alcohol and caffeine because they disrupt your mood with stimulants and depressants.

- Exercise daily to provide an outlet for stressful emotions and anxiety. Exercising releases endorphins which promote healthy moods.

- Spend time meditating and breathing deeply. A simple count to 10 while breathing slowly and deliberately can reduce anxiety and deliver a sense of wellbeing.

- Eat a balanced diet because the natural nutrients in a balanced diet are necessary for maintaining a healthy mood.

- Learn to recognize what triggers your anxiety so you can take action before you become anxious.

Depression is different from anxiety, lack of motivation and long periods of low mood and lack of interest in everyday activities can easily trigger sleep disturbances, both too much and a lack of sleep are common.

The following tips can help anyone to cope with the symptoms of depression and this can help promote a healthy restful sleep.

- Reach out and stay connected to family and friends. This can be difficult when dealing with depression, but pushing yourself to do it anyway will boost your mood and reduce the feelings of guilt you may have over neglecting close relationships...just do it.

- Exercise, it will release endorphins and give you a mood boost. Choose exercises that are continuous and repetitive like riding a bike or using a treadmill.

- Use meditation, simple meditation practices can improve your mood, practice breathing with focus, breathe in and exhale purposefully and focus on it as you do.

- Don't skip or skimp on meals, a healthy diet will support a healthy mood.

There are many ways to fight depression including medications and talking with your doctor. These tips are meant to help you boost your mood before going to sleep.

A calm, relaxed mood will help you maintain healthy, beneficial, sleep habits. A refreshing, healthy sleep will also give you a mood boost to start your day and help keep you feeling relaxed, and refreshed.

Chapter 4 – 7 Steps to Break the Insomnia Cycle Forever

These 7 steps to break the insomnia cycle forever will change your life. It is important to give each step the time and focus it deserves so you can get the most from it.

These steps are not a quick fix; they require some work on your part. Once you begin, stick with it, breaking the cycle of insomnia requires life style changes and dedication.

Each step is designed to change the way you think about sleep and sleeping. Behavior modification is the best way to make changes that will stick and become part of your daily routine. As you progress through the steps you will begin to realize how life changing this process is.

As your behavior changes and these steps become part of you daily routine, insomnia will become something you can change, rather than something you struggle with or cope with.

Insomnia is more common in women than it is in men. Everyone responds to circadian rhythm. The circadian rhythm is what determines your wake and sleep cycle, it is attuned to the light/dark cycles in nature. When your circadian rhythm is out of sync, you will experience insomnia.

Insomnia can be short term or long term, both will respond to behavior modification and the steps in this chapter. Remember, these steps are meant to help you change your behavior and thoughts about sleeping. Changing how you think about sleep, think about where you sleep, and the routine you follow as the day winds down will make an impact on your life, and break the insomnia cycle.

Step 1

Regular Sleep and Wake Up Times

I know what you are thinking, "how can I establish regular

sleep and wake up times if I am experiencing insomnia!", well

there is an answer for that.

Snapping your fingers and announcing when you will go to bed and when you wake up is not going to establish anything; changing how you think about sleep can.

Interestingly enough, our thoughts can actually change the way we think and behave. Setting a time to go to bed and a time to wake up will help reset your circadian rhythm and help you on your way to meet the sandman.

Establish a time to go to bed that will give you at least 8 hours of sleep before you have to wake up for work.

The time you set is symbolic as well as a command for your subconscious to focus on. Once you have a sleep time that you are happy with, decide on a wake up time.

As you decide on a wake up time, think about how much time you woul

d like to have before you have to leave for work. Give yourself enough time to wake up and start your day without rushing or starting off stressed.

Your sleep and wake times must be thought of as an essential part of your daily routine, these times are as important to your wellbeing as the meals you eat and the job you perform at work or school. You must put positive thought behind these times that you have chosen, and you must tell yourself just how important they are.

These positive thoughts about sleeping and waking will eventually take hold in your subconscious and help you in your battle against insomnia.

Think about it, you probably already have a round about time to go to sleep and it probably stresses you because you know you are not going to be sleepy or you have brought your work home with you and you are stressing about completing it before you turn in.

You probably also have a slew of negative thoughts and emotions about waking up. You stress about not hearing the alarm clock, not getting enough sleep before the alarm goes off...the list is endless.

All of these negative thoughts about going to sleep and waking up make an impact on your subconscious and eventually on your circadian rhythm.

Now, choose two good times, times that provide you with a full 8 hours of sleep and time to wake up and start your day stress free, no rushing!

Do not stress about anything that involves your sleep time or your wake time; this may be tough at first, but things will fall into place.

The next step is going to help you stick to your established sleep and wake times without causing you any anxiety or stress.

Step 2

Prepare for Sleeping

This is a very important step, preparing for sleep will become a routine, and routines are behaviors that help you get things done the way you want them done.

Routine is repetition, repetition becomes habit, and habit paves the way for behavioral modification that will either benefit you and your agenda or not.

The point is, you are going to be in control of your behavior and the results; no more wishing or complaining, it's time to be doing.

Preparing for sleep involves creating a routine that helps you relax, grow sleepy, and go to bed ready to fall off to sleep.

Your routine will involve positive thoughts, emotions, and associations that will put you in the mood to fall asleep.

This preparation routine will change how you think about going to sleep, and how you feel when you climb into bed.

Make a list of things you like to do that help you relax. Maybe reading a book, a relaxing scented bath, some meditation, or a hobby you enjoy. As you create the list, write down how you feel when you think about these relaxing things.

Write down your thoughts and emotions next to the things that help you relax. Now set aside at least an hour for engaging in one of these things each night before you turn in.

This hour you have set aside is probably the most important change you are going to make. When the time arrives to relax and enjoy personal time before bed don't let anything get in the way.

Read what you wrote about how this activity relaxes you and gives you a peaceful moment during your day. Don't leave out the part about reading what you wrote, it is important to reinforce the positive thoughts and emotions associated with this activity. The next step will support this step and help you stick to the routine.

Step 3

Make Your Bedroom a Sleeping Paradise

Where you sleep can really change your sleep life. Take time and create a space that is dedicated to sleep and sleep only (and sex of course). No TV in the bedroom, this may be a difficult thing to come to terms with but there can be no TV watching in sleep paradise.

This list will help you create your ultimate sleeping paradise:

- No television in the room

- No computer in the room

- Decorate with calming colors, nothing distracting or stimulating

- Pay attention to textures, colors, and patterns in your bedroom

- Keep the room cool, it is easier to sleep in cool temperatures

It is important not to watch television or work/play on the computer in the bedroom. Keep the room dark when you sleep, light can affect the natural circadian rhythm. If you room gets light from neighbors, street lights, or road lights, try room darkening shades/curtains to keep the light from disturbing you.

Artificial light, especially blue light, they type of light that comes from televisions and computers disrupts melatonin production. Melatonin is a hormone involved in regulating sleep. Amber tinted glasses have been proven to reduce the amount of blue light to your eyes; wearing these glasses at night before bed can reduce the amount of blue light and keep it from suppressing melatonin production.

Keeping the room cool can actually help you fall asleep. When the body begins to get ready for sleep, it begins to release heat from the core to the skin and into the environment. If the room is too warm, this process is slower to work and this can contribute to insomnia.

Step 4

Exercise and Natural Light

Add an exercise routine to your daily routine. If you already have an exercise plan or are just starting one now, make sure some of the exercise takes place outdoors.

Natural sunlight during the day will help regulate your circadian rhythm. Exercise itself is known to contribute to sleepiness at night; the more exercise and light you enjoy during the day, the better chance you will have at getting a goodnight sleep.

Your circadian rhythm is a delicate cycle, getting proper amounts of sunlight, and darkness will help regulate your inner clock and this will help you fall asleep and stay asleep.

One of the best ways to reset your circadian rhythm is to go camping. Camping and exposure to natural light and dark schedules will reset your inner clock and get you back to sleeping every night.

Step 5

Diet Changes

There is no need to change everything about your diet to help relieve insomnia. Adding some carbs to your dinner will naturally help you fall asleep. Carbs release tryptophan and this induces sleep.

If you are on a low carb diet, your diet could be contributing to your insomnia.

It is no good to eat large amounts of food before bed or drink excessively before bed. Eat at least 4 hours before bed, this gives the body time to digest before you turn in.

Adding some carbs to your last meal will release tryptophan slowly into your system and by the time you are ready for bed, you will feel naturally sleepy.

Do not eat carb laden food right before bed, eat it during your last meal to give the carbs a chance to break down and help you fall asleep.

Alcohol is a remedy everyone talks about but it is not a remedy, it is actually the enemy. Drinking alcohol before bed may get you to sleep faster than normal but it will also wake you up.

Alcohol will stimulate you and wake you up several time during the night, and this is no way to get a refreshing sleep. Eliminate alcohol and add a few carbs; this will help you sleep and stay asleep

Step 6

No More Stimulants

Remove all stimulants from your diet, this may be tough, but it will improve your sleep. No more coffee or drink decaf coffee; coffee, no matter what time of day you drink it, can have adverse effects on your sleep. Caffeine lingers in the system and can really wreak havoc with sleep.

Caffeine is in more than coffee, it is found in cola drinks, and other soft drinks so read the labels, it is in tea of all types, unless it is decaffeinated, and stay away from chocolate, chocolate has caffeine in it too.

Removing stimulants from your diet will help you regain a natural sleep wake cycle. This won't happen overnight, but it will happen. Continue using the other steps while removing stimulants from your diet and natural sleep cycles will return.

Replace those caffeine drinks with water; water is important for keeping body systems regulated, dehydration can creep up on you and it causes leg cramping, another sleep killer.

Step 7

If You Do Not Fall Asleep Get Up

If you follow all of these steps you will begin to notice a natural sleep cycle returning. While you are practicing these steps, this step will be an important one.

If you do not fall asleep within a half an hour get up. This may seem counter intuitive for someone with insomnia, but believe it or not, it will help.

Get up if you cannot sleep and leave the bedroom. Remaining in bed and trying to force yourself to sleep will only cause frustration and stimulate your thoughts; it is better to get up.

Try going to another room and reading from a book, not a digital book, a regular book; a digital book emits blue light and this light is stimulating. Try and relax and read a book or magazine, anything that is calming, nothing that will wake you up.

Once you feel tired again, go back to the bedroom and try to go to sleep again.

If All Else Fails

The steps in this book will return your natural circadian rhythm and you will once again enjoy a good night's sleep. If these steps do not work as they should, there is another alternative, seek cognitive therapy.

Cognitive therapy will address the reasons you cannot fall asleep. Sometimes there are reasons you cannot relax, and if stress is keeping you awake regardless of your best efforts, a cognitive therapist can make a difference for you.

Cognitive therapy is about learning behavioral techniques that will help you conquer your insomnia. The steps in this book are very similar to behavioral techniques but working with a cognitive therapist is one step better. Insomnia is something you can defeat, and if you need a little extra help relaxing, a cognitive therapist will help.

Another big factor for those with insomnia is health. Remember health problems can trigger insomnia; and some medications can also trigger insomnia. As discussed elsewhere in this book, be sure you don't have any underlying health problems that could be causing your insomnia.

Conclusion

Your new outlook on how to conquer insomnia will serve you well and help you get the sleep you need. Remember, some steps may help you more than others, it all depends on your specific insomnia and its cause.

Don't give up, continue the steps, it will work; it is similar to the way behavior modification works.

Regular restful sleep is attainable and you have taken the initiative to make it happen for you. While nothing is perfect, getting the sleep you need is really a matter of making the changes needed and sticking with them.

Now you have information that will give you the tools to take action and end the struggle forever.

While the steps in this book will work to release you from the grip of insomnia, you should still see a doctor and get a medical diagnosis of your condition.

There are many health conditions that can cause insomnia; insomnia itself can be a side effect of a health condition so before you use the steps in this book, see your Doctor for a diagnosis.

www.ingramcontent.com/pod-product-compliance
Lightning Source LLC
Chambersburg PA
CBHW070241290526
45789CB00004B/1711